I0787866

Alkaline Diet

Volume 1

By Ryan Ball

Copyright 2017 - All rights reserved.

This document is geared towards providing exact and reliable information in regards to the topic and issue covered. The publication is sold with the idea that the publisher is not required to render accounting, officially permitted, or otherwise, qualified services. If advice is necessary, legal or professional, a practiced individual in the profession should be ordered.

- From a Declaration of Principles which was accepted and approved equally by a Committee of the American Bar Association and a Committee of Publishers and Associations.

In no way is it legal to reproduce, duplicate, or transmit any part of this document in either electronic means or in printed format. Recording of this publication is strictly prohibited and any storage of this document is not allowed unless with written permission from the publisher. All rights reserved.

The information provided herein is stated to be truthful and consistent, in that any liability, in terms of inattention or otherwise, by any usage or abuse of any policies, processes, or directions contained within is the solitary and utter responsibility of the recipient reader. Under no circumstances will any legal responsibility or blame be held against the publisher for any reparation, damages, or monetary loss due to the information herein, either directly or indirectly.

Respective authors own all copyrights not held by the publisher.

The information herein is offered for informational purposes solely, and is universal as so. The presentation of the information is without contract or any type of guarantee assurance.

The trademarks that are used are without any consent, and the publication of the trademark is without permission or backing by the trademark owner. All trademarks and brands within this book are for clarifying purposes only and are the owned by the owners themselves, not affiliated with this document.

Table of Contents

Introduction

In the beginning, let me thank you for purchasing the "**Alkaline Diet Vol 1**" book!

There is a bunch of different diets available to you these days, and it's hard to select the perfect ones. When you think about the best way of nutrition, it should be the one that has the most advantages, especially in the long-term. That is exactly what alkaline diet is as it provides you with everything you need to live a healthy lifestyle which will secure the perfect balance of your body.

Here is what we will cover in this book:

- **Alkaline diet overview** – all the necessary information you need to know about this way of nutrition, including its origin and primary principles
- **Why alkaline diet is your best choice** – all health advantages of alkaline diet and how it can benefit your overall health
- **Complete food guide to alkaline diet** – the most comprehensive part of the book that will secure you all the info required to know about foods you need to avoid and limit during the alkaline way of nutrition. We will also discuss eating out and nutritional supplements while you are on this diet

- **How a day on alkaline diet looks like** – a practical example of a day of your alkaline lifestyle should look like, from the morning until you head to sleep. Includes an example meal plan suggestion
- **Preparing to start** – valuable insider tips that will make the beginning phase of your alkaline diet a whole lot easier. We also list the most frequent mistakes people make in the starting period so that you can be aware of them in advance

Let me thank you once again for purchasing the Instant Pot Ketogenic Diet Cookbook. I hope you will enjoy reading it!

Alkaline Diet Explained

The alkaline diet is one of the best ways of nutrition you can choose if you are looking to make a transition to a healthy lifestyle that will not only help you shed extra pounds but also assist you in leading a healthier life and eating high-quality food.

Scientific research relates the development of various illnesses to how our digestive system works, and how it subsequently influences the immune system of our organism. You can imagine that your digestive system is nothing else but a filter. We use it to filter the micronutrients and other ingredients from the food we consume. But what happens when we put unnatural ingredients, such as preservatives or additives, into this filter? It has trouble to process them, and the result is that it gets clogged. That, in turn, can lead to numerous health issues in our organism. Fortunately, there is a fantastic way of nutrition that will keep your digestive system from clogging – the alkaline diet.

What Is Alkaline Diet

The alkaline diet is a way of nutrition that promotes consuming foods that are believed to influence the acid-base homeostasis in the organism. Bluntly put, it is a diet that promotes eating raw organic vegetables and fruits for one simple reason – they produce an alkaline effect and help your body maintain the alkaline environment. Keeping your body's environment alkaline has a number of benefits, including boosting the immune system, increasing energy, and helping you lose weight.

To understand how alkaline diet works, we need to see what influence your body's pH levels can have on your overall health. Let's take a closer look at what exactly is pH we just mentioned.

PH is a figure expressing either the alkalinity or acidity of something. The scale starts at 0, which marks that something is completely acidic, to 14, which marks that something is entirely alkaline. The middle of the range (7) is a neutral zone. For example, pure water is known to have a pH of exactly 7. Next, sulfuric acid is extremely acidic and corrosive and has a pH of close to 0. Lye is on the other hand of the scale and has a pH level of almost 14. However, lye is as corrosive as sulfuric acid, but for whole other reasons – it is highly alkaline.

As for the human body, if it is going to function properly, it needs to have its pH maintained in a narrow range – from 7.35 to 7.45. According to research, the bodily fluids and tissues have the perfect working environment in that pH range. That doesn't go for stomach, which has a pH level of 3.5 and we need it to stay that way so that it can properly break down food. On the other hand, blood has a neutral pH value because it has the role of transporting different substances from one place in our organism to another and it needs to do that without reacting or influencing them in any way.

Problems can occur when there is an imbalance of pH in an organ or system. In fact, if your internal pH levels incline too much toward being completely acidic or alkaline, the consequences could be fatal. Yes, it also means that it's not good to have a too alkaline body. The key lies in the balance.

How the Alkaline Diet Works

Believe it or not, the full name of the alkaline diet is "balanced alkaline-acid diet." As you can see, the primary focus should be on balancing your internal pH levels. Your body always strives to keep its pH levels at the narrow range that it considers the perfect environment (between 7.35 and 7.45).

The goal of the alkaline diet is rather simple – it needs to keep the balance between acidity and alkalinity in your body. Considering that Western cultures today have a way of nutrition that promotes highly acidic foods, alkaline diet concentrates on promoting different kind of food that will help you achieve the pH balance.

According to experts who have been studying and recommending the alkaline diet for years, the ratio you need to stick to is 80:20. That means that you are allowed to eat only 20 percent of foods that are considered highly acidic once you begin this way of nutrition. On the other hand, the majority (80%) of your food should come from the foods that are considered alkaline-promoting, such as vegetables.

Let's take a look at some foods that are believed to be alkaline forming:

- Garlic
- Avocado
- Mustard Greens
- Apple Cider Vinegar
- Pumpkin Seeds
- Almonds
- Green Tea

Making sure that you eat 80% of alkaline promoting food will ensure that you keep the pH balance of your organism. That way you can take advantage of multiple positive effects, including losing body weight and boosting your overall health.

Does It Work?

The question that concerns most people is, does the alkaline diet work? The short answer would be – yes. This way of nutrition works, and it is recommended by doctors around the world, especially for patients with certain conditions, such as the ones attending chemo.

After all, the alkaline diet is based on sound principles that are approved by various health authorities and nutritional experts around the world. They all agree that fruits and vegetables have a positive effect on the overall health of a human being, and veggies and fruits are the focus of the alkaline diet. That means that you can't go wrong if you decide to change towards the alkaline way of life – you can only make your body healthier.

Can You Keep Track of Acidic Levels in Your Body?
Not only you can do it, but it is pretty affordable, and you can do it in less than 30 seconds. The only thing that you need is a test strip that measures pH level you can buy in a local pharmacy.

However, measuring your pH level only once is not going to provide you a reliable result. Instead, you should look to track your pH for at least several days (preferably a month).

There are three tests you need to perform during one day:

- **Morning saliva test** – use the strip to test your saliva right after you wake up. That means that you should do it before brushing your teeth or drinking any water. The level should be somewhere between 6.9 and 7.3

- **Morning urine test** – measure the pH level of the first urine of the day by using a pH test strip. The level should also be between 6.9 and 7.3.

- **Second urine test** – it is desirable to check the second urine before having breakfast (if that is possible). You can drink water or green tea in the meantime. The level should ideally be between 7.35 and 7.45, but certainly around those numbers

If the tests show you that you incline toward having acidic internal pH levels (lower than 7), you could definitely use a change in nutrition, which makes you the perfect candidate for the alkaline diet.

The History behind the Alkaline Diet

When you take a closer look at the history of the nutrition of the humanity, you come to one simple conclusion – the food we eat today is almost entirely different to the one our ancestors used to eat. First of all, our early ancestors mostly consumed raw food that was plant based and they ate meat only on rare occasions.

However, modern technology made changes to both how we get and prepare our food. We use refined and processed grains today, and we use a lot of salt to add extra flavor in our food, compared to some earlier periods when salt was only used a bit in veggies. An even worse the thing is that the evolution of humanity enabled it to pick up the pace of growing animals. Meat has become one of the main ingredients of nutrition in the Western cultures. The same goes for dairy products, which are something that the early humans never consumed. There is no need even to mention that the sugar consumption has increased numerous times. Changing the food we eat also caused the humanity to make the transfer from alkaline toward acidic diet.

Alkaline diet has been the subject of scientific studies for decades. Physiologists, in particular, studied what influence it has on urine acidity, as well as the role the kidneys have in body's mechanisms to regulate the acidity of bodily fluids. Claude Bernard, a French biologist, conducted a research where he observed a group of rabbits whose diet he changed from mostly plant (herbivore) to mostly meat (carnivore). The diet modified the urine and made it more acid than before. Subsequent research led him to discover that metabolizing different foods might leave different traces in human organism (acidic foods leave acid marks, and alkaline foods leave alkaline traces).

The hypothesis made by Bernard was under the careful analysis of nutritionists at the start of the 20th century. At the time, they emphasized the roles that cations (positively charged particles) and anions (negatively charged particles) have in our diet. They came to a conclusion that sulfate, phosphate, and chloride are acid forming, while magnesium, calcium, and potassium are alkaline forming. The interesting thing was that the first group of elements consists of anions and the second are all cations. They also discovered that particular food has particular effect on pH of the urine.

As for the historical use of the alkaline diet, it was used to keep kidney stones from reappearing. Due to its ability to affect pH of the urine, the diet was also used to prevent recurrent urinary tract infections.

Why You Need Alkaline Diet

The alkaline diet promotes pH balance in your organism because it is the ideal environment for it to work properly. The problem with today's Western styles of nutrition is that they include highly acidic foods, which can cause a bunch of problems to our bodies.

After all, what do you think of when somebody says acid? I bet that it is nothing good. Well, that's right – acid can make holes through metal, which means that there is nothing positive it can do to your tissues, muscles, and digestive system. Some acid is needed for our organism to work, but too much can easily lead to health issues.

You can measure if your internal pH levels are highly acidic by using test strips, but you can also listen to your body because it might be giving you signs that you should change something.

How to Notice if Your Body is Too Acidic
- Here is how your organism might manifest poor pH balance:
- You feel tired all the time, even when you've had a good night sleep
- You don't feel like you are in a mood to do anything and you have trouble enjoying things that used to make you happy
- You have trouble with concentration, and you can't seem to focus on anything
- Your brain often becomes "foggy."

- You find that you are irritated for no apparent reason
- You experience headaches frequently
- You have joint pain often
- Your neck frequently feels sore or stiff
- You have sensitive teeth and gums
- You often experience diarrhea or constipation, and you can notice that your digestive system doesn't work properly
- You frequently have flu, colds, and infections
- You have problems with your skin, such as acne

If you can relate to more than one thing on this list, there is a good chance that you suffer from pH level imbalance. An alkaline diet can help you deal with this problem and solve the health issues you might have. In fact, let's take a look at multiple benefits of the alkaline diet when it comes to your health.

Health Advantages of Being on Alkaline Diet
It Can Protect You from Cancer

The study conducted in The Great Britain concluded that there is more chance that your body will kill cells that carry cancer if you keep your internal pH levels balanced. Sticking to the alkaline diet can improve your immunity and therefore help you prevent the risk of cancer appearing. Furthermore, the alkaline diet is what the doctors recommend to patients that are already undergoing chemotherapy because it increases chances that it will work.

How Alkaline Diet Increases Immunity

It works like this - if you want to get rid of body waste, you will need to have an adequate level of minerals in your cells. Insufficient amount of minerals results in reduced vitamin absorption, and it is the reason why toxins and pathogens can easily hit our immune system and weaken our overall health.

Arguably the most important mineral you need to have in your body is magnesium because it is among the primary reasons why various processes in our organism work properly. The deficiency of magnesium can cause headaches, muscle pain, sleep deprivation, and issues with cardiovascular health. On the other hand, magnesium improves vitamin absorption, especially vitamin D, which is integral to our immune and endocrine systems.

Keep Your Bone Density and Muscle Mass

This also brings us to securing your body a sufficient amount of minerals. That is crucial for your bone density and muscle mass. There are numerous studies that confirm that alkaline forming foods decrease the risk of sarcopenia, decreased the strength of bones and muscle mass as you age.

Magnesium, phosphate, and calcium are among the minerals you want to lean on for keeping your muscle mass. That can help you prevent osteoporosis and other diseases that attack your bones.

Decreases Chronic Pain and Inflammation

Scientific research leaves no room for guessing –
being on alkaline diet helps you reduce chronic pain
and inflammation. The results of a study from Europe
with 82 participants noted significant pain decrease in
76 cases, which is over 90%. That means that you can
deal with chronic headaches, muscle spasms, back
pain, joint pain, and inflammation, simply by keeping
your hands of the highly acidic foods and achieving
the pH balance in your body.

Helps You Have Healthy Gums and Teeth

When your internal pH levels are highly acidic, the
organism will steal minerals to neutralize that acid. It
won't choose where it takes from, which means that it
will also take them from your mouth. The problem
occurs because the amount of minerals in one's mouth
is not that high. That is why tooth and gum decay are
among the sure signs of mineral deficiencies.
Furthermore, processed foods can swiftly create acid
that can corrode your mouth. So, if you are looking to
keep your teeth and gums healthy, you should make
sure to consume a lot of alkaline promoting foods.

Helps Removing Acid Reflux

Believe it or not, a study conducted in the United
States confirmed that 50% of Americans have trouble
with acid reflux. An alkaline diet can help you regulate
this because it contains no processed grains, sugar,
and other unhealthy food that decreases the

production of stomach acid (in this case, stomach acid is good, unlike the body acid).

Helps Your Skin Look Younger

Alkalization helps you deal with any skin problems you might have. That includes acne, eczema, rosacea, and psoriasis. Believe it or not, they have one common denominator – acid. These problems happen because your body is trying to deal with the excessive levels of acid and does that through the skin. Perspiration is one of the four ways our organism releases toxins. Regardless of how it manifests on your skin, it probably begins with what you eat, and it is mainly related to processed grains and sugar. Cutting them from your diet should greatly diminish your chances of skin problems and make your skin glow.

You Will Sleep Better

If you are waking up constantly in the middle of the night, that might be related to the fact that your body is overly acidic. You see, our organism is typically most acidic between 1:00 and 3:00 AM, so if you are waking up around that time, it might be a sign that your body is struggling to detoxify from acid.

Alkalizing your body during the day is the right way to secure yourself a deep and healthy REM sleep during the night. Kale, spinach, and Swiss chard can particularly assist your liver to detoxify. Another thing to make sure is to have the last meal in the day at least 3 hours before you head to bed. You can also think about taking a boost of potassium, calcium, and magnesium about half an hour before you fall asleep.

You Will Have More Energy

A study confirmed that if your hydration level decreases by only 5%, your energy levels can subsequently reduce for up to 30%. Whenever you feel like you lack energy, try the simplest 'solution by dilution' and drink some water. The alkaline diet promotes drinking at least eight glasses of water each day and, if you are looking to add some flavor, you can throw in a bit of lemon juice.

It Helps You Lose Weight

Extra pounds are also related to being overly acidic, which is why alkaline diet can help in two cases. The first one is if you are looking for a way to keep your ideal weight and the other is if you are seeking to shed a couple of pounds and reach the perfection when it comes to looks.

It's quite simple – most of the acid forming foods not only diminish the fat burning capacities of our organism, but they also influence that we feel hunger more often. On the contrary, foods that promote pH balance and alkalinity allow you to feel full after consuming them and without overeating. That is how alkaline diet can help you achieve the ideal weight.

Complete Food Guide to
the Alkaline Diet

Okay, we have not reached perhaps the most important section of our book about the alkaline diet. This chapter will teach you what foods you are allowed to consume and which you should avoid while you are on this way of nutrition. You will also learn how to handle eating out with your friends and make it fit with your diet, as well as how to use nutritional supplements to your advantage. Finally, there is also a meal plan suggestion so that you can get the idea how a day on the alkaline diet looks like.

The PRAL Scale

Although it doesn't really roll off your tongue, the PRAL scale is extremely useful in the alkaline diet. PRAL marks the level of alkalinity or acidity that a particular food has. That means that we don't just categorize food as alkaline or acidic, but we rather check the PRAL rating and see whether it is alkalizing or acidic and to what extent.

PRAL measures food's alkalinity or acidity based on the level of protein, minerals, and phosphorus that it leaves behind after being metabolized in our body. If it leaves traces of magnesium, calcium, and potassium, it is considered alkaline promoting, while leaving phosphoric and sulfuric acid means that it is considered acid forming. With that in mind, let's take a look at the food you should eat and avoid on an alkaline diet.

Foods You Should Eat

In short, the foods that are considered most alkaline on the PRAL scale are veggies and fruits, as well as several seeds and nuts. Here is the list of foods that needs to find its way into your diet.

Beet Greens

According to the PRAL scale, beet greens are the world's most alkaline food. They might not be the most popular one in our way of nutrition but think about adding them to your stir-fries, smoothies, salads, or soups. They can replace any other green, but beware – they do have a bit of a bitter taste, which is actually good because it helps stimulate the production of bile which helps digest fats in a better way.

Spinach

Spinach is extremely rich in calcium, making it an internal ingredient that can help the health of your bones. Aside from that, it has a bunch of cleansing juices that help your organism detoxify and therefore can help prevent cancer. The good news is that there are a bunch of ways to be creative when preparing spinach and it is the perfect ingredient for smoothies.

Kale

I know that meat lovers might roll their eyes now, but kale is the new beef. It is rich in calcium, iron, and vitamin K, and can help you prevent cancer. Aside from that, its mild taste makes it a perfect fit with any recipe. Whether you want it in a salad, stir-fry, or soup, you can get a fantastic boost of alkalinity with kale.

Swiss Chard

I believe that you have noticed that we've listed only leafy greens so far. That's right; they are the world's most alkaline food and, as such, should be the integral ingredient of your new way of nutrition.

As for Swiss chard, it is also incredibly rich in vitamins, particularly vitamin K, which we already mentioned is important for preventing cancer. Aside from that, it has plant protein and phosphorus, but it doesn't make it an acidic food. The reason for that is that there are far more minerals that are considered alkalizing in Swiss chard. If you haven't so far, you can try using Swiss chard instead of a tortilla in any recipe.

Bananas

Bananas are known to be rich in fiber, which is essential for your digestive system and detoxifying your gastrointestinal tract. Yes, bananas are also rich in fructose (fruit sugar), which is why people who have weight issues avoid them. However, bananas will always be a far better choice than, for example, a granola bar or other acid promoting food.

Sweet Potatoes

Sweet potatoes are highly alkaline foods, but they are also rich in starch, which means that you need to consume them in moderation. Their PRAL score makes them an alkaline food, and they can provide your body with a boost of minerals, vitamins, and fiber. The fact that they are rich in fiber means that they don't impact the sugar levels in your blood too much because it's fiber that assists in slowly releasing the sugar into the bloodstream. That means that sweet potatoes are great when you are looking for an energy boost, but make sure to keep it moderate.

Celery

Celery is integral for the alkaline diet because of its cleansing properties. The high amount of water in it helps our body detoxify quickly. Aside from that, celery is an incredible ingredient for any diet because of the negative calorie index. That means that the calories you spend chewing and digesting is higher than the amount of calories celery itself contains.

Carrots

Your parents might have told you to eat a carrot when you were little because it will help with your eyesight. That's true, and the reason is high vitamin A content in carrots. Believe it or not, just a cup of carrots contain three times the RDA (recommended daily amount) of beta-carotene, which is a form of vitamin A. Aside from helping with your eyesight, it also promotes the health of your skin and makes it younger-looking, and it can play a role in preventing cancer.

Kiwi

Kiwi is another type of food rich in minerals, vitamins, and antioxidants. Somehow, oranges became famous for the amount of vitamin C in them, but the truth is that there is for times as much of vitamin C in kiwi. Aside from that, the fiber it contains help with digestion and potassium will help with the proper function of your muscles.

Cauliflower

Women whose estrogen levels are elevated should consume cauliflower because it can help with rebalancing the hormones. It is achieved through Indole-3-Carbinol, which is a nutrient that helps in regulating estrogen levels in our body. You can have elevated estrogen because of the estrogenic foods (soy), oral contraceptives you have been drinking or even chemicals in your vicinity (plastics, for example). Higher estrogen levels can lead to extra pounds, as well as cause bloating and even infertility and reproductive cancers. Cauliflower can significantly help in regulating your estrogen levels.

Cherries

Another fruit on our list of alkaline promoting food is cherry. They have a plethora of antioxidants that can help in protecting against cancer. Aside from that, they are related to protecting cardiovascular health, and they can play a role in relieving you of pain linked to arthritis and joints. Cherries are an excellent addition to smoothies, but you can also consume them as a snack.

Eggplant

Eggplant brings some healthy phytonutrients into your organism, such as chlorogenic acid. Although it is called acid, it actually helps with metabolism and digestion because it is a plant compound. Eggplant is an excellent addition to salads, and you can also bake it in your oven.

Pears

Pears are among the fruits that have low sugar content, making them an excellent choice even for those who are having trouble with imbalanced levels of blood sugar. They are also high in fiber and vitamin C, which plays an integral role in protecting against cancer.

Hazelnuts

Hazelnuts are one of the rare nuts that have an alkalizing effect. They are a fantastic substitute to highly acidic peanuts and the right choice for a snack.

Pineapple

Believe it or not, you can find pineapple in some of the nutritional supplements, which should be enough to witness its positive effect on human body. The reason why this is the case is bromelain, which is a digestive enzyme that kills intestinal parasites and boosts digestion.

Zucchini

Zucchini is needed in your alkaline diet because of lutein, which is an antioxidant in the same category like beta-carotene. That means that it can play a role in keeping your eyesight unhindered. Zucchini is also an integral ingredient of various low-carb diets, and it can be a great alternative to pasta.

Strawberries

The immunity system mostly benefits from vitamin C you can find in strawberries. Aside from that, they contain manganese which aids the metabolism of our body. Strawberries are a perfect addition to smoothies, and they can be used in various desserts.

Apples

An apple a day keeps the doctor away. While the saying might not be entirely correct, apples are still extremely healthy for human body. They are rich in vitamin C and antioxidants called flavonoids, which boost immune system and help to prevent cancer.

Aside from that, they have a high amount of fiber which our body uses to detoxify.

Apples are also essential if you want to keep your cholesterol levels and blood pressure in order. You can also use apple cider vinegar, which also has advantages, such as acetic acid (a nutrient, despite its name) that has antiviral and antibacterial benefits.

Watermelon

Watermelon provides our body with potassium and other electrolytes necessary for cardiovascular health. It also assists in hydrating our body because it has a high amount of water (just like the name suggests). You can get creative and make a watermelon smoothie, or you can eat this fruit as a snack.

Raisins

If you have a sugar craving, raisins might solve that. They are full of antioxidants, and some studies even conduct that they can regulate blood pressure.

Garlic

There are people who claim garlic is a miracle food, and I can tell you that they are not wrong. It can boost your cardiovascular and immune systems, cleanse your liver and regulate blood pressure.

Lemon

Just like orange, lemon is famous for fighting flu and colds. These stories are entirely accurate as lemons truly fight viruses in our organism. Besides, they also can heal wounds, energize liver and help the body detoxify.

Cayenne peppers

Cayenne peppers have a high amount of vitamin A, as well as other antibacterial benefits, which are important for fighting stress and various diseases. Aside from that, they assist that endocrine function of our body works correctly.

There is not much wisdom when it comes to the alkaline diet. The food that needs to be in the focus when you are on this way of nutrition is fruits and vegetables. Although we listed some of them that have highest alkaline values, you can also consume other veggies.

Water

There is an ongoing debate whether alkaline water is truly useful or just bogus. It does have a higher alkalinity level than tap water or bottled options, but the health advantages are still to be confirmed. Either way, water is your go-to drink when you are on an alkaline diet, whether it is alkaline or pure. Sparkling water isn't such a great idea and heading for the tap is always a better option.

Tip: If you are looking to add flavor to your water, feel free to add some lemon juice.

Foods You Should Limit

Now that we've learned what should be our priority when on an alkaline diet, let's take a look at what food we should limit or completely avoid if we want to stick to this way of nutrition. All of the foods listed in this section have high acidic value. That usually means that you don't have to avoid them always and at all cost, but keep in mind the 80:20 ratio we mentioned in the chapter overviewing the alkaline diet.

Fruits and Veggies

Yes, there are some fruits and vegetables that have high acidic value, and that is why they are not recommended to eat when you are on an alkaline diet. As for fruits, you should limit blueberries, currants, and cranberries. The same goes for glazed and canned fruits which you should look to avoid altogether because they, in most cases, have artificial preservatives and sweeteners added. Another thing to bear in mind is that processed fruit juices also are highly acidic.

When it comes to vegetables, you should know that lentils, olives, winter squash, and corn all have high acidic value. They still have some nutrients and fiber, but you should look to limit their use in your nutrition plan.

Dairy

Bad news for all you guys and girls who love dairy – its use should be restricted in the alkaline diet. You might wonder why that is the case since they are rich in calcium, but the truth is that the acidic value trumps the benefits we get.

Unfortunately, it won't make a difference if you choose low-fat versions of dairy. The only right thing to do is to severely limit products such as various cheeses, yogurt, milk, and butter in your nutrition. The same goes for eggs, especially for yolks, which also have high acidic value.

Grains

The thing with grains is that baking and processing destroys the good things we can get from them and turns them into products that are overly acidic. Add to that the fact that they have an insufficient amount of nutrients and fiber to offer and that is enough to stay clear of these products.

Grains that you should limit include white bread, pasta, doughnuts. bagels, pastries, biscuits, crackers, and white rice.

Meat

Yes, meat can be an important source of proteins, but there is one thing to bear in mind – once the protein is metabolized, it is considered acidic. The reason for this lies in purines, the compound that forms uric acid. That not only has an acidifying effect on our internal pH levels, but it can also spread to joints and tissues and cause issues such as kidney stones and gout.

That doesn't mean that you should avoid meat at all costs. Remember the 80:20 ration in favor of highly alkaline foods and make sure that you always pick free-range and organic meat because they have a higher amount of nutrients.

Nuts and Oils

If we are on the hunt for a protein source to include in our nutrition, nuts are a much better option than meat and other animal products. The reason lies in the fact that they are not as acidic as meat once metabolized. However, most of them (except hazelnuts) still have an acidifying effect which means that you need to eat them in moderation.

As for oils, sunflower seed and canola oil, just like other vegetable oils, have a moderately high acidic value. That also doesn't mean that you should avoid them altogether, but you should keep their use moderate.

Refined Sugar

We've now come to an item that is a big no-no in the alkaline diet (and in any other healthy nutrition plan). Processed sugar is extremely acidic and is one of the primary reasons why people even have elevated internal pH levels in the first place. The body needs to work hard to neutralize the acidifying effect of processed sugar, and there is no reason to put it through that trouble.

Completely avoid muffins, sodas, candy, pastries, and other foods that are considered to be "leisurely."

Coffee

The users of coffee will be disappointed with this item on the list. All forms of coffee are overly acidic, but if you really need to allow yourself an occasional cup or two, make sure that it is something like Swiss water decaf, which has lower overall acidity.

Alcohol

Regardless of the amount of calories it has, alcohol is strictly forbidden in the alkaline diet because it is overly acidic. It will steal essential minerals like magnesium from your body and can also generate stomach aches if you are sensitive to overly acidic foods.

Here are some other tips you can use when it comes to foods to limit and avoid during alkaline diet:

- Make sure to stay clear of food preservatives and artificial sweeteners and coloring. Any food that contains these ingredients should be avoided since it is considered extremely unhealthy
- Avoid using antibiotics or drugs at all (except when medications are prescribed by the doctors)
- Avoid swallowing your food quickly. Instead, find time to properly chew it to additionally decrease the acidity of the body

Eating Out Guide

I still haven't met a human being who doesn't occasionally enjoy eating out. The reason might lie in the social factor because eating out usually means that we will get together with some friends and have a fun time. When you start your alkaline diet, you might face certain challenges to stay on the right track when eating out. That doesn't mean that you should steer clear of hanging out with your friends. If you read the tips we've got prepared for you, there will be no trouble to eat in a restaurant and keep the balance of your internal pH levels.

First of all, you need to do some research before you head out. You can think ahead and research the restaurants in your area that are considered to be the healthiest. Alternatively, look at the menus on their websites and choose the main dish that suits your alkaline lifestyle in advance.

Another important thing to bear in mind is that you shouldn't be hungry when you go to the restaurant. That way you will be under more temptation to try some of the overly acidic food there. A good way around this is to simply have a light snack before you head out.

Once you arrive at the restaurant, order a salad with leafy greens. That will secure two things – you will boost your alkalinity levels, and you will feel full sooner. There is no need to feel an obligation to order the main course, too. You can choose two appetizers instead. For example, after you finish the salad you can ask for a vegetable soup.

If you do order an entrée, salmon might be an adequate choice. Make sure to ask if the fish is fresh and whether it is wild or farmed (the first option is better). Naturally, you should avoid eating anything fried, as well as grains, including the bread that the waiter might bring to the table. Be aware that restaurants often allow you to choose the sides, which means that you can pick vegetables or leafy greens.

As for the dessert, consider skipping it altogether. The reason lies in the fact that desserts in the restaurants are usually full of refined sugar and high in calories.

When it comes to drinks, herbal tea and water are a much better alternative than sugary beverages, which you should avoid. The same goes for coffee, but if you have to drink it, try to limit yourself to one cup.

Here are some other tips you can use when eating out:

Don't hesitate to communicate with the waiter. After all, he should be aware that he could get a generous tip if he tries to answer all your questions and fulfill all your requests. In case he was nothing but kind to you, make sure that you thank him with an appropriate tip

You can always ask one of your friends to share a dish. That is a good way to control portion size and eat less

Ask the waiter to bring you condiments on the side. That way you can control how much dressing you want in your salad and make sure that you will avoid any unhealthy stuff, such as mayonnaise

Take time to chew your food – just like you would to at home, enjoy the experience and eat your meal slowly

Stay away from salt – in most restaurants; there is salt on the table in case you want to add some extra flavor to your dish. However, these are usually not healthy salt options, so it might be best to avoid it

Nutritional Supplements

Nutritional supplements can help you in keeping your body slightly alkalized, just like the alkaline diet requires. Although you are eating a bunch of healthy food, there are some supplements that can help you on your way toward making your body more alkaline.

We will list some of the supplements that people on the alkaline diet most often use. However, it might be a good idea to consult with your doctor or a health professional before you include them in your nutrition.

Green Powder

These powders usually contain a combination of chlorella algae or spirulina and juices of wheat, barley, or alfalfa grass (in most cases, a mixture of everything listed). When you take a look at the ingredients, you might get a feeling that you will drink something that reminds of swamp water. However, if you dilute it in a cup of water or even in a smoothie, you will be pleasantly surprised at how tasteful green powders are.

As for their health advantages, they will boost the alkalinity of your body and therefore provide you with extra energy and improve your immune system. A bunch of different green powders is available on the market, and you will surely find the appropriate test for you. However, make sure that you chose a reliable manufacturer that got good reviews.

Calcium

When your body's internal pH levels start leaning toward the acidity, the organism begins withdrawing minerals from everywhere, including your bones. If your bones suffer regular calcium losses, they will become vulnerable. Calcium is one of the minerals whose supplements can be valuable to your bone structure and density. As for the daily range, it varies from one person to another, but the RDA (recommended daily amount) is between 800 to 1500 mg.

Magnesium

In the case of acidity, the same thing that happens to your bones also happens to your muscles. The only difference is that magnesium keeps your muscle mass and strength. Believe it or not, the research shows that 3 out of 4 people suffer from lack of magnesium. If you often suffer from muscle tension or headaches, try to look for the cause in magnesium. Using mineral supplements might be helpful. The recommended daily amount is between 400 and 800 mg.

PH Powders and Drops

Aside from the classic supplements, there are specially designed formulas whose goal is to help balance your internal pH levels. They are on the market by the name "pH powder" or "pH drops" or something like that. These powders and drops usually have a solution of hydrogen peroxide or chlorine dioxide, which has the ability to release oxygen in your organism and that way it enables to restore the ideal pH levels. Aside from that, these supplements can also contain minerals, such as calcium, magnesium, and potassium.

The problem is that the quality largely varies depending on the manufacturer or the ingredients. When choosing pH powders or drops, try to conduct the research about the manufacturer and read the label carefully.

That concludes the list of supplements that are recommended for use during the alkaline diet. We once again remind that you shouldn't start taking any new supplements before consulting with a health professional.

A Day on the Alkaline Diet – Meal Plan Suggestion

If you've carefully read the book up to this point, you know which foods you can eat and which you should avoid when on an alkaline diet. But how a day on this diet actually looks like?

That is an interesting topic that deserves a closer look. Let's see how a day when you apply the 80:20 ratio in favor of highly alkaline food looks like. Before we start, keep in mind that you don't have to adhere to these suggestions strictly. The alkaline diet is flexible, but you should find some useful guidelines here that will assist you in getting off the acid quickly and correctly.

Waking Up

There is a good technique you can use in the morning that can help you reduce your stress levels. It has a bunch of positive sides, including the fact that it helps regulate blood pressure, slow down your heartbeat, and energize the muscles. However, the most significant advantage is that it can adjust your internal pH levels.

The technique is simple – you should inhale through your nose for about 3 seconds. The next step is to hold your breath for about 6 seconds and then you should exhale through your mouth for 5 seconds. Aside from using it in the morning, feel free to apply this technique whenever you find yourself under stress.

Exercising

It's not a bad idea to exercise in the morning as it will give you the energy needed for the upcoming day. About 15 minutes is more than enough to get your blood pumping and increase your heart rate. You can use a mini trampoline called a rebounder, which is a highly useful way of cardio exercise and can help you lose extra pounds even more than running. Of course, if you can't afford or you don't have a rebounder, running is also a good investment.

Breakfast

In most cases, your breakfast choice should be a proper smoothie. The things that you should include in your smoothie are low-sugar fruits, such as avocados, leafy greens, as well as some healthy fats like hazelnuts, flax seeds or chia seeds. You can also add almond milk, coconut milk or even coconut water (pure water can also be an option).

Of course, there are other options for breakfast on the alkaline diets, which include gluten-free oats combined with fruit, or even a mix of quinoa, strawberries, and chia seeds.

Morning Tea

A couple of hours after your breakfast you should have a morning tea to help you stay hydrated. An excellent idea might be detox tea, which has a lemon, ginger, cayenne, and turmeric. Green tea is also an incredible choice, but the thing to avoid is coffee. Naturally, you should also drink water whenever you feel the need to hydrate.

First Snack

In case you feel hungry before lunch, you can allow yourself an alkaline snack. For example, you can take some healthy alkaline mix full of raw almonds, hazelnuts, chia seeds, and sunflower seeds. Alternatively, prepare another smoothie and drink that. However, don't feel that you need to have a snack before lunch and only resort to this in case you are hungry.

Lunch

Sweet and savory salad or kale pesto pasta are fantastic choices for lunch. You can also have a nice hot vegetable soup. The important thing to remember, if you are preparing a salad, is to keep it colorful, which means that you should include as many different vegetables and fruits as you can.

Occasionally, you can allow yourself fish or meat for lunch. In that case, choose free-range and organic animals or fish full of healthy protein such as salmon.

Afternoon Snack

The middle of the afternoon is a good time for the second snack of the day. Good choices are something like hummus sticks (or other vegetable sticks) or kale chips. The important thing is that you keep to snacks that have little or no sugar and little protein. If you have sugar cravings in the afternoon, try that, and you will see that you will resolve the issue!

Working Out

After you are done with your job, it might take me a good time to exercise again. Running or simply walking is an excellent way to unwind. About an hour of activity should be enough. Bear in mind that you have to hydrate; make sure to drink enough water during the entire day.

Dinner

As for dinner suggestions, you can prepare a vegetable mix or whip up another salad. Alternatively, you can make quinoa bowl and, depending on the amount of protein you've consumed during the day, you can also include their healthy form in this meal.

Dessert

It doesn't have to be mandatory, but if you were a sugar addict, there are alkaline desserts that can help you once you make a transition to the alkaline diet. For example, the chocolate avocado mousse is an excellent way to go, as well as chia pudding. One thing to make sure is that you have this dessert at least 2 or 3 hours before you head to bed.

Final Notes

Nutritional supplements are not mentioned here, but you read in the previous chapter that you can and should include them in your alkaline diet. The use of supplements should be in accordance with the instruction manual on their box, but if you only have one dose during the day, aim for it to be in the morning or after lunch.

Finally, this is just a suggestion on how to lead an alkaline way of life. It's hard to make a 100% change at once, which means that you don't necessarily to try to stick to everything that was written in this chapter (at least not during the first days of your diet). I will mention once again, the essential thing to take into consideration is that your nutrition should consist of 80% alkaline promoting foods and that is the primary rule of the alkaline diet.

Preparing to Start

We are making some real progress – you know now much more about the alkaline diet and how your meal plan and lifestyle should look like if you want to stick to it. However, experience teaches us that the hardest thing is to start a new way of nutrition and successfully pull through the starting phase until you get accustomed to your diet. Some research indicates that it takes about three weeks to change your habits and make the transition to a new lifestyle. You will have to go through many temptations in this period so let's take a look at some tips that might help you on the way.

Tips to Prepare for the Alkaline Diet
Keep It Simple and Start Slowly

The reason why many people give up when they are starting a new diet is that they are making a transition too difficult for both their body and mind. If you were a fan of acid forming foods, making a complete change towards alkaline food at once might be troublesome.

You should allow yourself a couple of weeks to develop healthier habits. During this period, you don't have to burden yourself too much. Try to have a strong will and follow as much of the guidelines we mentioned in this book as you can. However, don't be too harsh on yourself and, in case you make a mistake, don't dwell on it. The right thing to do is to move on and concentrate on getting back on the right track as soon as possible.

Physical Activity Matters

Perspiration is one of the four ways our body releases toxins, which is why sweating matters. The best way to sweat healthily is to exercises. Running and other cardiovascular exercises (we mentioned rebounder) are fantastic. However, if you are just a fan of walking, try not to skip spending at least an hour in the local park and walk for at least several miles each day.

Stay Hydrated

Hydration is an integral element of every diet, and alkaline nutrition is no exception. Your goal is to drink at least eight glasses of water every day. Precisely, your objective should be half of your body weight in ounces. That means that if you weigh 150 lbs. you should drink 75 ounces of water each day.

If you are looking for extra flavor, add some lemon juice or even some apple cider vinegar to your water.

Green Smoothies Are Pure Gold

Smoothies are an incredible mix of vegetables and fruits packed with healthy nutrients and can be an excellent boost to your energy, especially in the morning. Each of your smoothies should by default include some leafy greens (spinach or kale), a banana or small amount of berries of your choice and maybe even some healthy fats, such as chia seeds.

Prepare Your Meals in Advance

Believe it or not, this is the second most frequent reason why people abandon a diet plan. When you think of it, preparation is integral to any particular way of nutrition. Just imagine – you just came home after spending a whole day at work. You see that there is nothing for dinner and the weather is cold and rainy for you to go to the store. In that case, ordering a pizza or grabbing that unhealthy snack from the cupboard seems like an excellent choice. Another moment passes, and you've already threw away your diet for some convenient unhealthy food.

When you are cooking and preparing alkaline promoting meals, make sure to cook for a couple of days in advance. Salads can last for several days if you keep them in the fridge and the same goes for most of other dishes. Aside from that, make sure that you have enough of raw ingredients in the fridge that you can quickly whip yourself up a meal whenever you feel like it.

The tip that nutritional experts provide is that you always need to know what you will eat at least two days in advance. That might not necessarily include preparing that food, but you need to have exact ingredients for that recipe in the fridge. By avoiding shopping impulsively or on a day-to-day basis you can allow tiredness or hunger to control what groceries you will buy and that is not a good thing for your diet.

Eat Regularly

Another important thing to remember when on an alkaline diet is to eat regularly. It is a far better option to eat more often in modest amounts than having one large meal. Not only it will stress your digestive system, but it will make you hungry again quickly. Splitting your meals evenly across the entire day is a way to secure that you won't feel hunger and, even if you do, you can always deal with it by having a healthy fruit snack.

Enjoy Your Meals

Our digestive system has trouble taking large pieces of foods, and premature swallowing can lead to more acid being created in your body. The digestion process begins in our mouth when we start chewing our food. While we are chewing, essential enzymes that help the digestion process are released. By making sure that you have enough time for a meal, you ensure that you won't stress your digestive system.

Treat every meal as a time for relaxation. A convenient way of controlling your chewing is that you shouldn't reach for your fork until you make sure that you have completely chewed and swallowed what is currently in your mouth. Besides, alkaline diet offers a bunch of extremely healthy and tasteful meals, and there is no reason not to savor them.

Mistakes to Avoid in the Beginning
You Neglect Breathing Exercises

We mentioned that you should do deep breathing exercises each morning and any time when you feel under stress. There is a reason why experts recommend this; it is a great way to regulate the level of carbon dioxide and expel the excessive amount through respiration. Next time when you think about skipping breathing exercises, try remembering that carbon dioxide is 100 times more acidic than other acids in your organism COMBINED.

Don't Look for Quick Weight Loss Results

If one of the goals of your alkaline diet is to reach your ideal weight, you will need to be patient. After all, the alkaline nutrition focuses more on changing your lifestyle and making your overall health significantly better. That also goes in line with regulating your weight, but nothing happens overnight.

After the first week on the alkaline diet, you will certainly notice some progress, especially because you won't feel bloated like you did before. As time goes, you will realize that you are making constant progress and that all it takes is a little patience.

And the best news when it comes to the alkaline diet and weight loss is that – once you reach your ideal weight, alkaline diet secures that you will keep that weight for a long time because it is a long-term nutrition plan you can stick to by the end of your life.

You Kept Unhealthy Snacks

As soon as you start your new way of nutrition throw away (or give as a gift to your neighbors or friends) all unhealthy snacks that you didn't eat up to that point. If you have on your mind that there is a snack in the cupboard, it is far more likely to tempt you and lead you to break the rules of your diet.

Don't Be Afraid of Acidic Food

While there are things that you should completely avoid (we mentioned them in the food guide in this book), it doesn't mean that you should be afraid of having some acidic food, especially if it can secure your protein and other nutrients. After all, we learned that balance is the key to the alkaline diet. As long as you are sticking to the 80:20 ratio, there is nothing you should worry about.

Risks and Concerns

Alkalosis Explained

If you remember, we mentioned in one of the previous chapters that alkaline diet has a full name "alkaline-acid balance diet." As already told, the goal of this way of nutrition is to achieve and maintain the balance of base and acid in your body. That is done by maintaining pH levels. The modern Western way of nutrition often puts your body into acidosis which, although it is mild, can cause damage to some organisms. The same goes another way around – it won't do anything well if your body becomes too alkaline either.

Human body's ideal internal pH levels are between 7.35 and 7.45. Considering that seven is considered as a neutral number on acid-alkaline pH scale, that means that you should keep your body slightly alkaline to keep it healthy. However, if your alkalinity reaches an abnormally high level, that's a sign of a state called alkalosis.

What Causes Alkalosis?

One of the reasons for the alkalosis is following an extremely high alkaline diet. If you keep to 80:20 ratio, that is something that happens rarely, but you have to be aware that there is a small possibility of that occurrence. Aside from that, alkalosis can be caused by excessive vomiting, which makes us lose hydrochloric acid, as well in case of severe diarrhea.

Alkalosis can be developed by a significant increase of bicarbonate or a sudden drop of carbon dioxide. There are five types of alkalosis, including hypokalemic, hypochloremic, compensated, metabolic, and respiratory alkalosis. The symptoms and causes for each of them can significantly vary, and the severity of the condition can also vary.

What Are the Symptoms?

In most cases, you will first experience confusion and feel light headed, which might lead to fainting. Other symptoms include muscle spasms, tremor in the hands, numbness or tingling in the face, vomiting and nausea and shortness of breath. Alkalosis can also lead to irregular heart beat also known as arrhythmia.

What Is the Treatment?

The treatment depends on the type of the acidosis in question. If you do feel that you have multiple symptoms from the upper list, the best way to do is to consult your doctor. There is a way to quickly help yourself by grabbing a paper bag and breathing into it as that can contribute to restore the level of carbon dioxide in your blood and lower its alkalinity. However, medications are the quickest way of correcting the pH imbalance, so make sure to check in with your health provider immediately.

Other Concerns

There are no other pressing concerns related to alkaline diet aside from severe pH imbalance.

Conclusion

That concludes "**Alkaline Diet**" books. Thank you for reading it!

I surely hope this book was of great help in understanding the alkaline diet in a better way. The goal was to explain everything related to this way of nutrition understandably. We covered all areas of the diet, including a complete food guide and how to prepare to start your new alkaline way of life. The only thing left now is to be persistent as it is a fire-proof way to make the transition to alkaline lifestyle.

Finally, if you enjoyed this book, then I'd like to ask you for a favor, would you be kind enough to leave a review for this book on Amazon? It'd be greatly appreciated.

Visit the link below to leave a review:
https://www.amazon.com/review/create-review

Thank you and good luck!

www.ingramcontent.com/pod-product-compliance
Lightning Source LLC
Chambersburg PA
CBHW050759240726
48654CB00008B/560